This to Me

Dr. A.H.Yurvati

This to Me
Copyright © 2024 Dr. A.H.Yurvati

ISBN: 979-8991704847 (sc)
ISBN: 979-8991704854 (e)

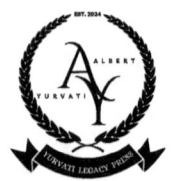

Yurvati Legacy Press
www.yurvatibooks.com
info@yurvatibooks.com

Table of Contents

This book is dedicated to the love of my life, Sharon. We are approaching our fiftieth anniversary in August 2024. I hope the Fates allow us to make that milestone. This is to my colleagues, residents, and students who have crossed paths with me. This is a special dedication to all the patients who entrusted me with their surgical care and recognition of two of my favorite patients. First was Norma Jean, who I saved multiple times because of ruptured arteries; she was my last case before I went into the hospital. Unfortunately, she passed away while I was recovering from my initial back surgery.

My second patient, Zakk, a musician from Colorado and founding member of the Broken Circle band, had a xiphoid issue that was inhibiting his life; he found me online and came to Fort Worth. We removed his xiphoid, and it was like a miracle; his recovery was rapid. He is now on the road, recording, and opening for some classical musicians. I foresee a Grammy in his future.

Acknowledgments

The author acknowledges Patrick Irish at the CVOR Medical City Fort Worth and his team for the cover photo; his talented artist, Melissa Gannon, who transformed the images into cover artwork; and Fulton Books, who helped him navigate the publishing experience.

Introduction

I hope you enjoyed my first book, *Wet My Hands*. I have been inspired by many of you to write another book. So here goes rubbish or not and my continuing saga with the dreaded Fates. Obviously, I am still alive from my initial diagnosis in 2010 of noncurable multiple myeloma. Many additional encounters with the Fates have occurred since our last interactions.

This is an update on Sharon. She required an urgent multilevel back surgery, in August 2010. We canceled our trip to Savannah at the last moment, as she fell in the bedroom due to loss of function in her right leg. She underwent a four-level laminectomy fusion and has made great progress with her physical therapist, Marc. Her expressive aphasia has not improved; we are now over three years from her initial stroke. Her fifth book of the Blood Moon series, *Winter Equinox*, has not been completed. The manuscript is on her Mac; I charge the device every month in order to save it. She was so close to wrapping up the saga of Candy and Thorne and their interactions with the Earth and Moon goddesses with the Sun god.

So with the permission of the Fates, let my journey commence.

Chapter 1

My adventure continues. I have had some major complications, and I will share those with you. I continued to have severe back pain, instability, and a restriction on my activities of daily living. I reconsulted with neurosurgery, and we determined that I needed a corpectomy (removal of the vertebrae and implant of a stabilizing device) of my third lumbar vertebra.

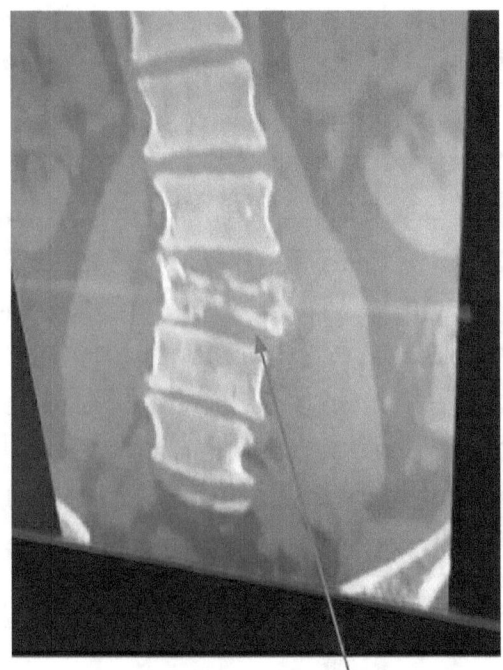

Arrow pointing to pathological fracture of third lumbar vertebra

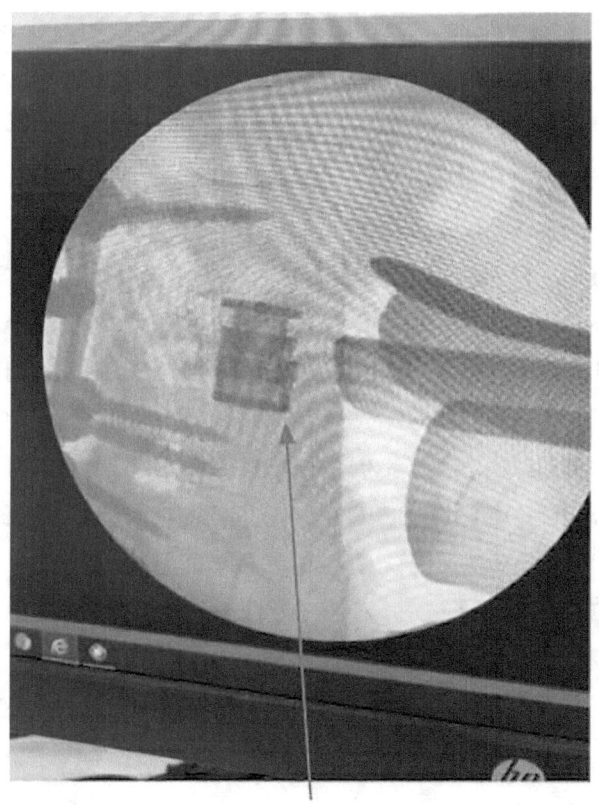

Implanted device

My second back surgery was extremely difficult; it was a ten-hour surgery. I spent one week in the neuro-ICU. I was incoherent, septic, and fluid overloaded and thought I would not make it. To make matters worse, the Fates hit me in the scrotum; major amounts of fluid cascaded downstream. My *cojones* looked like water balloons. After six weeks, I was walking without any assistive devices. Everyone thought I look great; then the Fates hit me. I had a sudden decline with my left sacroiliac joint subluxation (moved) trapping my sciatic nerve. Such severe pain is equivalent to my pain in 2010, so I'm back to a roller walker. To make things worse, I developed an acute superficial thrombophlebitis of my right ankle, my dominant leg. Such a mess in two limbs, pain, burning, and swelling. Talk about miserable.

Dr. Ash, my pain management provider, suggested an implantable pain pump, as he was hesitant to place pins in the joint in case they would not hold. So we did an epidural, and it was remarkable. He implanted a Medtronic synchronicity pain pump; the device has been a lifesaver, which allowed me to discontinue all opioids, and I feel so much more alert and alive. So here we go with another implantable device. I swear that when I am cremated, I will explode from all the batteries/devices implanted in me!

Chapter 2

We decide to celebrate my sixty-sixth birthday in Vieques, Puerto Rico. I asked Sharon's sister Vicky to come along to assist with her getting about. We left Dallas Fort Worth airport with an overnight in San Juan. I booked at the airport hotel; due to COVID-19, they had canceled then reopened reservations. Guess what? They lost ours! The hotel was full, so we spent the night in the lobby on chairs until our flight left for Vieques. It was only a twenty-plus-minute flight; all was going well, until we were preparing for landing. The landing gear would not deploy, so we aborted and returned to San Juan airport. The runway was prepared with fire trucks and emergency vehicles. The Fates! Luckily, the pilot was able to manually override and deploy the landing gear; we embarked for a short time and took another plane to Vieques.

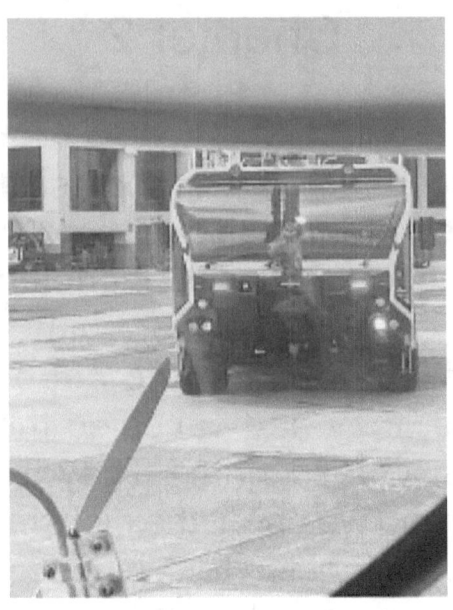

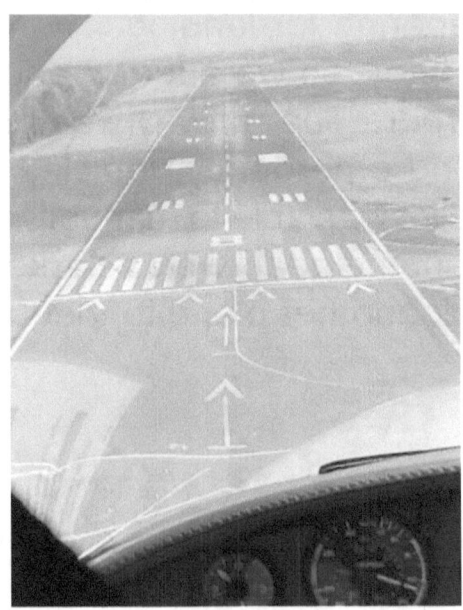

Upon arrival, we were greeted by my half-brother Jorge and his wife, Elba. I had not seen them in over forty years; it was an emotional reunion. We also met up with my nephew Jorge Alberto and niece Ive, who are fantastic people; my brother did a great job raising them; they are both successful. He built a vacation house up on a hill with a stunning view.

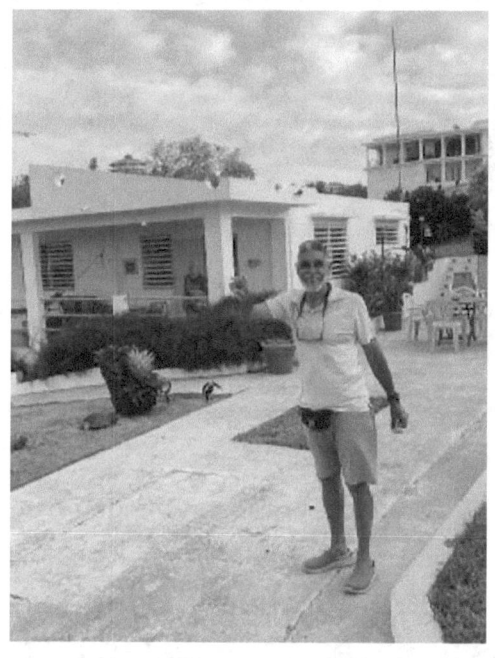

My brother's home in Vieques, which he built up on a hill overlooking the ocean, a view of Culebra, and a portion of the Virgin Islands

We stayed at the Blue Horizon Resort, in upscale bungalow accommodations, with a great view of the Caribbean Sea. Every day we would be picked up by family and taken to the beach; Sharon and Vicky were like fish, straight to the water. Our trip was very energizing.

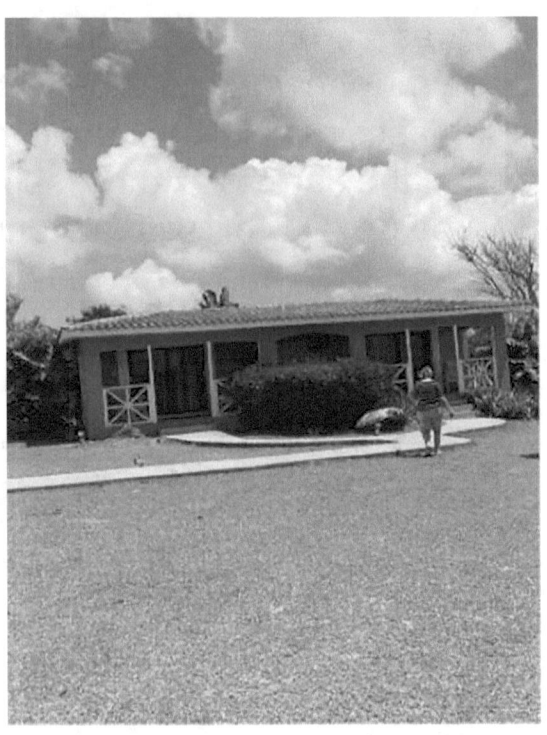

Blue Horizon Resort bungalow

We visited the area where my mother grew up; that part of the island was confiscated by the US Navy. The Department of Defense had started searching for a location to situate a naval base between 1941 and 1950, consisting of two parcels making up twenty-two thousand acres or about two-thirds of the island. Inhabitants were given a stipend of $1,500 to evacuate. Subsequently, eight thousand acres on the western end of the island was primarily used as a naval ammunition depot until the property was returned to the municipality of Vieques on May 1, 2001. The eastern end of the island was used for live training exercises, ship-to-shore gunfire, air-to-ground bombing, and US Marine amphibious landings starting from the 1940s onward. Within that area was a nine-hundred-acre live impact area (LIA) used for targeting live ordinances. Many areas are contaminated, and cleanup will take decades to decontaminate, if ever.

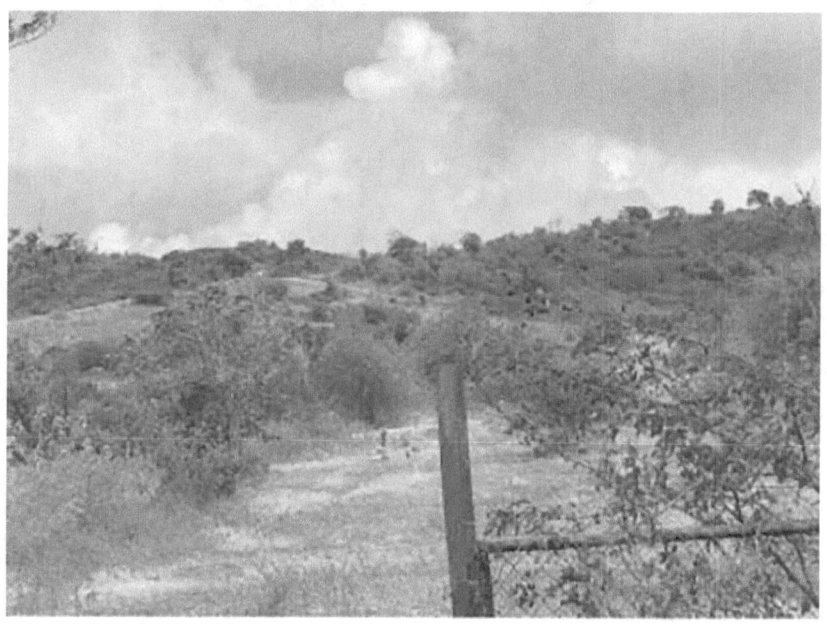

Family land, homes were razed by the Navy

An interesting thing about Vieques are the wild horses. Where did the horses on Vieques come from? This magnificent breed was cultivated over a period of five hundred years in Puerto Rico and is a blend of the Barb, Spanish Jennet, and Andalusian horses.

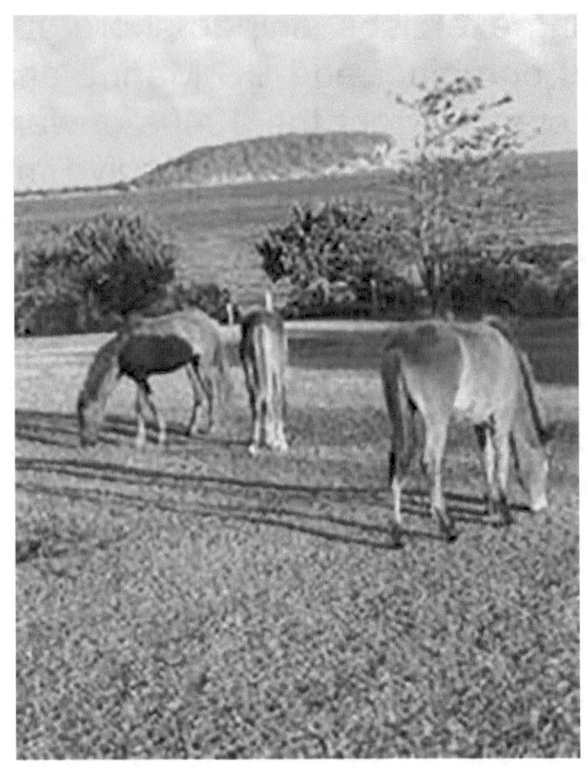

Wild horses

Another must-see sight is the ceiba tree. Ceiba trees, sometimes called kapok trees in English, dot the island, but there's only one known as the ceiba. It's the island's oldest tree, estimated to be upward of four hundred years old; the ceiba is the national tree of Puerto Rico.

It's easy to see why ceibas like this one occupy such a unique place in indigenous mythology. In Maya culture, ceiba trees marked the center of the earth, and the young branches covered in spikes like sharpened chainmail were believed to serve as a ladder allowing the spirits of the dead to ascend to the afterlife. In the religion of the Taino, Puerto Rico's indigenous people, the ceiba tree is considered the daughter of Yaya, the all-powerful goddess.

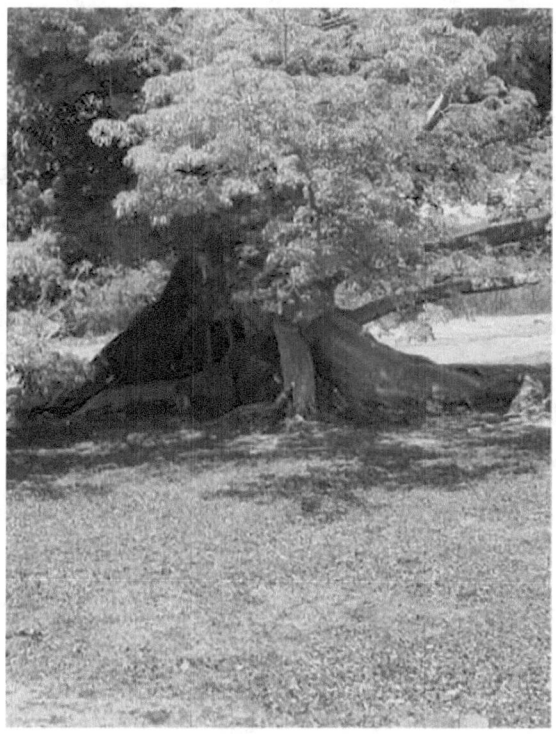

Vieques ceiba tree

Our return to the United States was uneventful; we actually had an airport hotel reservation, and our flights were on time. It was a very rewarding trip, reconnecting with family and experiencing the island my mother grew up on.

Chapter 3

My sixty-seventh birthday was much better than my sixty-fifth. We decided to do a road trip and invited Sharon's niece Lara and her husband, Geoff. We drove from Southlake to San Antonio (293 miles). We celebrated my birthday on the Riverwalk with dinner at *Boudros*. They have fantastic tableside guacamole and a signature prickly pear margarita. Our favorite accommodation is the Omni La Mansion on the Riverwalk; we always book a room with a balcony, such a gorgeous view. We did the obligatory riverboat tour, and I identified across the river at the Hilton La Placida hotel the table where Sharon and I had our first date in 1973.

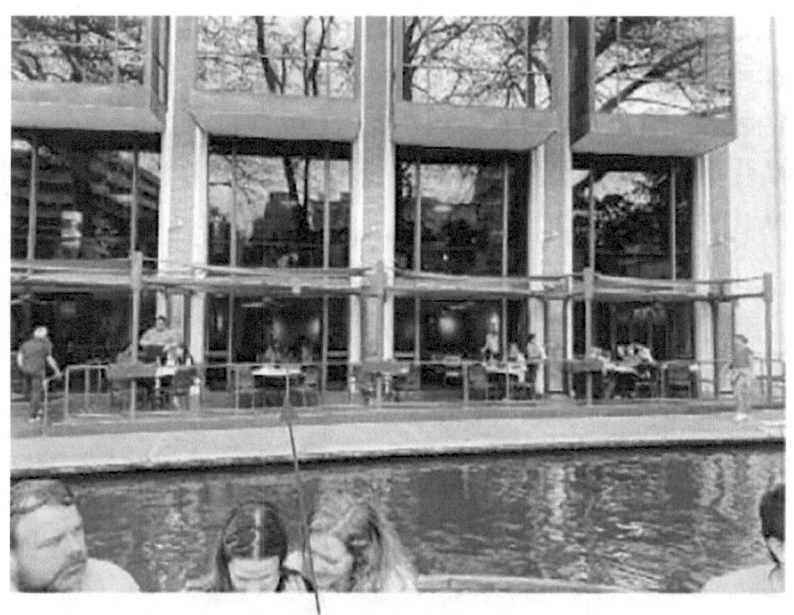

First-date table

The next day, south to Corpus Christi (145 miles), we stayed two nights at the Omni on the bay and visited Sharon's sister Vicky, who moved there and has a cute house on the canal. The final trip is to Fredericksburg (214 miles); we did wine tours and great dinners. Geoff's parents met up with us; they are retired naval officers. I saved my T-shirt: "ARMY because no one played Navy as a kid"; I did not want to start an Army versus Navy competition. Finally, we returned home (253 miles). It was a long road trip, 905 miles total, but was a great trip. The low back held up and needed some additional oral steroids but powered through the driving.

Coming home restarted chemo; all markers are holding steady, so we will remain on a maintenance schedule and hold bone marrow transplantation for now. The Fates have been very quiet; I wonder what they are planning.

Chapter 4

I was told by one of my attendings that in your surgical training, you think you have seen it all. Then he said it is not true: "*Once in practice, you will be presented with some unusual cases. That's why medicine is an art and science.*" I will present to you some of my most notable patients; I have attempted to explain the cases so nonmedical readers can understand what I am talking about.

I certainly miss going into the operating room, but with my condition, it's not possible; the privilege of helping someone, curing a disease, or saving a life is so uplifting. Many times you have to be innovative in your procedure; many times residents or students would ask me, "Have you done this before?" My answer is "No, no one has. You need to think outside the box."

I can recall my first and last surgical cases. My first was an eighty year-old woman, Mary, who sustained a left anterior descending coronary artery dissection during an angioplasty. To complicate the case, she had undergone in the early 1960s a Halstedian mastectomy (removal of the breast and all muscle) and cobalt radiation. Her chest tissue was like leather; it was a very difficult case. I did this on my own as my partner was out of town. She took forever to heal as expected. A year or two later, I operated on her carotid arteries, and years later, I bypassed her leg arteries.

My last case was Norma Jean. I had done aortic reconstruction twice on her and numerous lower extremity procedures, and she had a nonoperable pseudoaneurysm of her left iliofemoral artery. I would receive a message from her daughter that her mom was on the way to the ER via ambulance or care flight. I repaired the artery only to have it rebleed a few months later. She was the last case I did; I was in so much pain but felt committed to help her. I was recovering from my initial back surgery when her daughter informed me that she ruptured and was being flown in, but it did not look like she was going to make it. I was saddened, but I know I did everything I could to keep her alive to see her grandchildren and enjoy some family life.

So here we go back to the operating room so I can share with you some of my most unusual cases.

Chapter 5

Turtle Man

A fifty-one-year-old man was referred to our thoracic clinic with worsening shortness of breath, fever, and chills. His chest x-rays showed a collapse of the upper part of his right lung, with the formation of a bulla (bubble). His occupation was a bridge painter. He would clear out the birds' nests prior to painting; he did not comply with wearing protective respiratory equipment.

We took him to surgery and did an Eloesser flap; this is a procedure in which you take out some ribs and make a larger opening in the chest to drain. Three years later, he represented with multiple bacteria in his chest, most notably methicillin-resistant staph (MRSA). The best drug to treat MRSA is vancomycin. So I got the idea to make PMMA (polymethyl methacrylate) beads and place them in his chest. After a month, I removed the beads, and his infection finally cleared up. So how did I get the idea? Thinking outside the box. The chest x-ray shows the beads inside his chest. Thus, the image of turtle eggs!

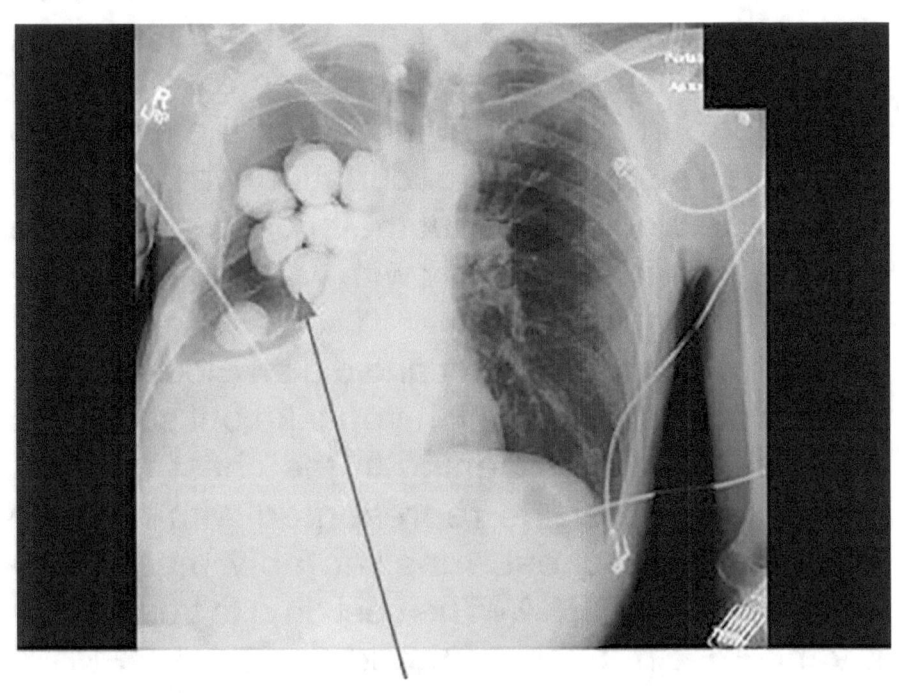

Methyl methacrylate balls with antibiotic

Chapter 6
Nail Lung

A forty-four-year-old psychiatric patient presented to the emergency room with a cough and hemoptysis (coughing up blood). He had a long history of swallowing glass, screws, nails, and other nondigestible items. He had at least four abdominal surgeries to remove the foreign bodies. A chest x-ray showed a nail in the left bronchus airway.

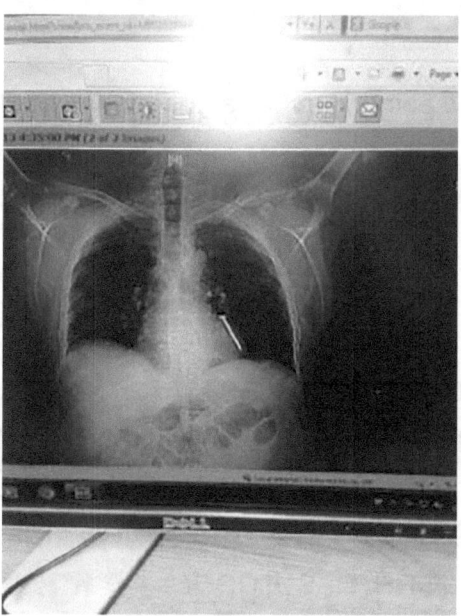

Pulmonary attempted to remove the nail with a bronchoscope but could not free up the nail. So cardiothoracic surgery was consulted.

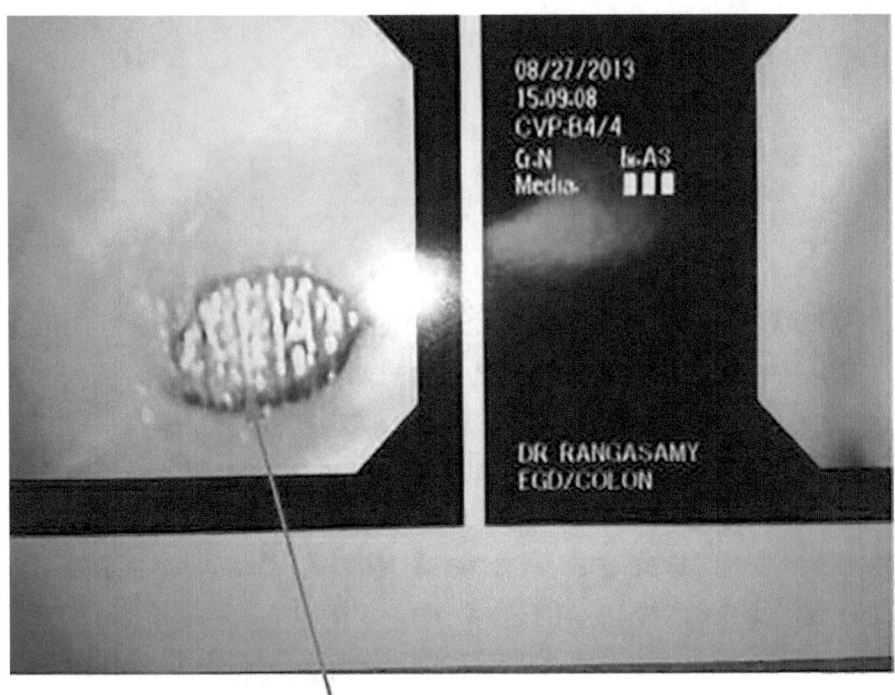

Arrow pointing to nail embedded in bronchus

We took him to the operating room and tried to remove the nail with a scope which failed. So we did a limited thoracotomy (open chest) and opened the lung to retrieve the nail. I stapled the lung close to preserve as much as I could. He did well and was discharged in three days. However, he returned a month later to the ER, this time with screws obstructing his intestine; luckily, I handed him over to general surgery.

Chapter 7

Hut Lung

An eighty-four-year-old frail Laotian woman presented to her primary care physician with fatigue, weight loss, and malaise. She immigrated to the United States five years ago; prior to that time, she lived in a small village. Hut lung or domestically acquired particulate lung disease (DAPLD) results from prolonged exposure to biomass fuel smoke causing an accumulation of anthracosis and fibrosis. Biomass fuel is used by greater than 50 percent of the world and includes wood, twigs, grass, charcoal, and other crops or natural residues. When burned, the smoke from the biomass fuel produces fine particles and dust, which settle in the bronchioles and alveoli. In the study by Sandoval et al., they discuss how wood smoke is composed of particles of varying sizes, "carbon monoxide, sulfur oxides, nitrous, oxides, aldehydes, and polyorganic matter, including polycyclic aromatic hydrocarbons," all of which are harmful toxins and pollutants that can irritate and damage the lung parenchyma. If ventilation is poor, there is an increased risk of inhaling these fine particles and pollutants, and over time, these particles accumulate and overwhelm the macrophages that normally rid the lung parenchyma of these foreign particles. Thus, the particles that are not removed by the macrophages can irritate the lung parenchyma and cause fibrosis or just remain in the tissue causing anthracosis.

We performed a right video-assisted thorascopic biopsy of her lung. The pathological diagnosis was hut lung; the picture shows the pneumoconiosis (trapped material in the lung).

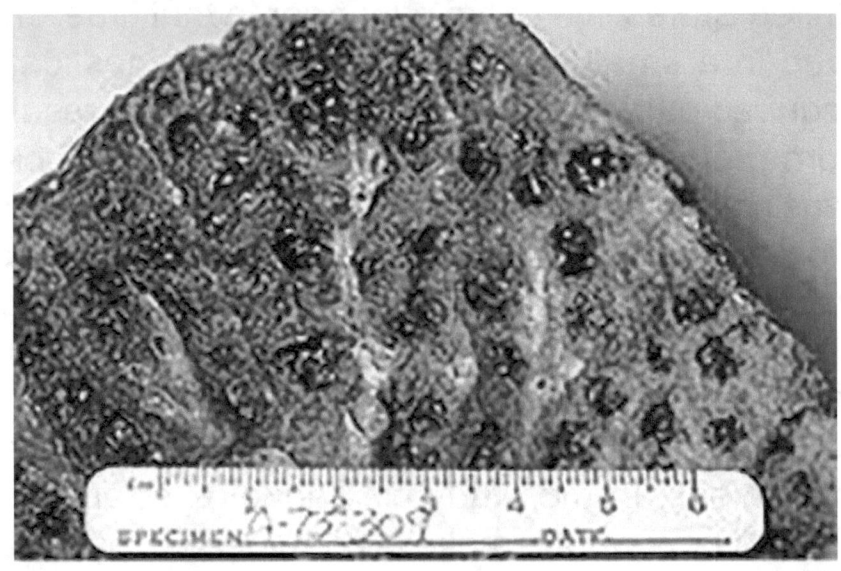

The patient was discharged in two days; unfortunately, there is no cure, and she continued to decline due to malnutrition and worsening lung function.

Chapter 8
Thoracic Spleen

A sixty-two-year-old woman presented to our clinic from her primary care physician with an abnormal CT scan of the chest. There was the appearance of a 3 cm. mass. We recommended video-assisted thorascopic (VAT) biopsy of the mass.

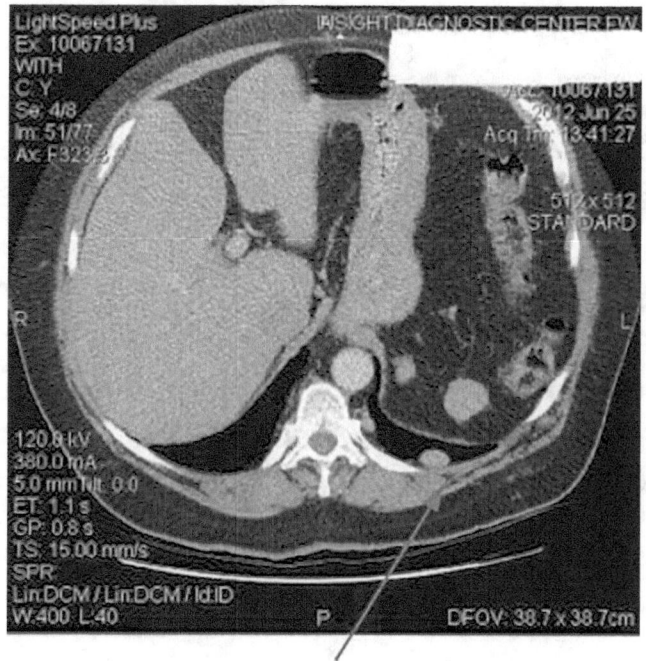

Arrow pointing to the mass

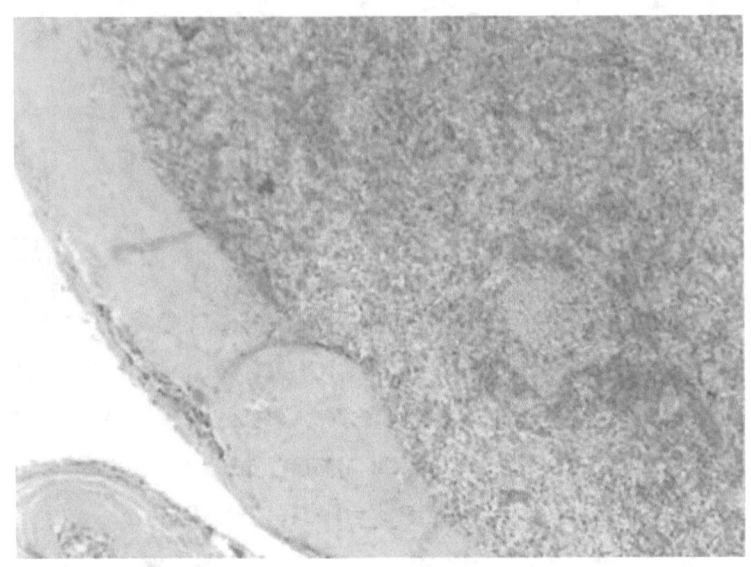

Splenic tissue

The mass was removed by video-assisted surgery, and pathology identified it as splenic tissue. Now, the spleen lives in your abdomen on the left side, not in your chest! Turns out that at age nineteen, she was shot at close range with a shotgun; we surmise a small bit of splenic tissue embedded in the chest and grew over time. Since 1856, only fifty-six intrathoracic spleen cases have been reported.

Chapter 9

Bilorrhea (Coughing Up Bile)

A forty-seven-year-old woman presented to the thoracic surgery clinic for a persistent cough, fever, chills, dyspnea, night sweats, and chest pain. She complained of a bitter-tasting yellowish fluid that she kept coughing up. Approximately one year prior to presentation, she had undergone a partial hepatectomy (liver resection) for a metastatic colon tumor. Post-op, she developed a lung infection and required video-assisted drainage. We diagnosed a very rare condition; a fistula (track) had developed between her liver and her lung.

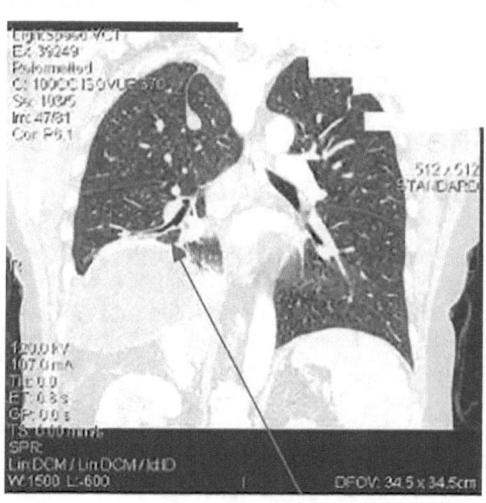

Arrow pointing to fistula

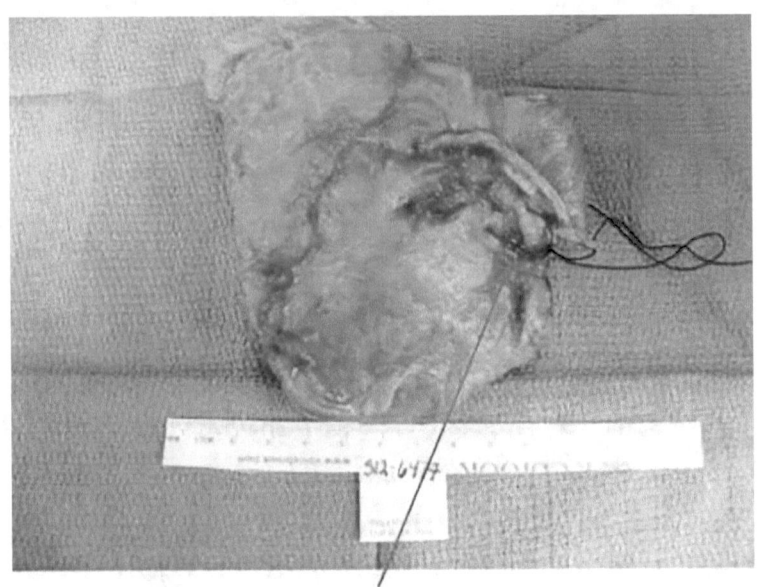

Arrow at suture where the fistula formed

She underwent an open resection of her lung to ablate the fistula. She was discharged in four days and did well. Unfortunately, her colon cancer came back, but she and her husband were able to go on a European vacation with no further coughing. She passed away about one year later from metastatic colon cancer.

Chapter 10

Intraparenchymal Lung Chest Tube

A seventy-four-year-old woman was visiting Texas from her hometown of Glasgow, Scotland. She was attending a family funeral in one of our rural communities. She had a history of COPD, lung cancer, and prior upper lung resection with radiation. She was short of breath and went to the emergency room; in the ER, they misdiagnosed a pneumothorax (collapsed lung) and attempted to place a chest tube. Unfortunately, they speared the lung and embedded the tube. She was helicopter transferred to our facility for surgical management. She was in shock and required urgent surgical intervention. We were able to remove the tube and stop the lung bleeding. This was a challenging case due to her prior surgery and radiation. We were able to suture the holes close and used surgical glue to seal, and she was stable post-op.

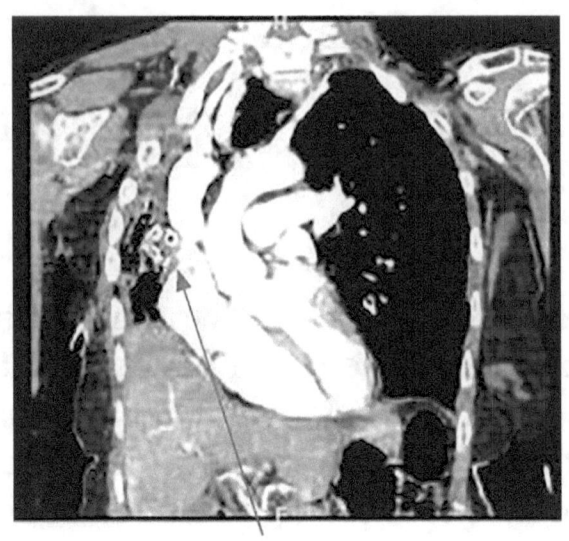

Arrow pointing to chest tube embedded in the lung

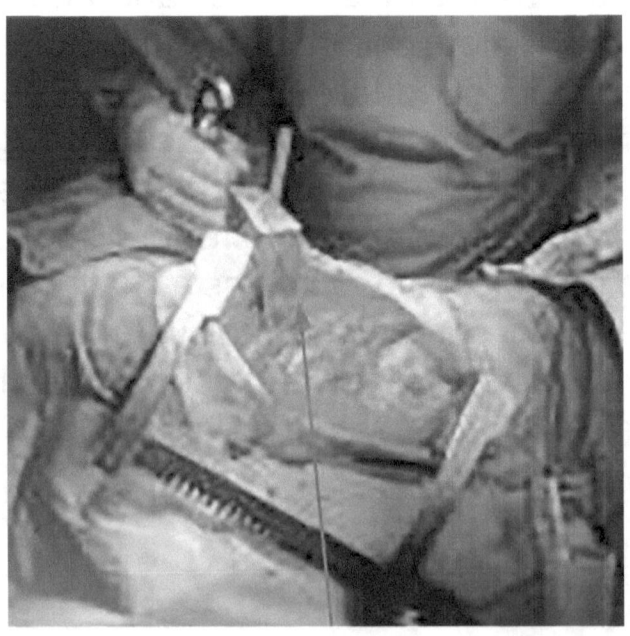

Arrow to operative exposure of the embedded chest tube

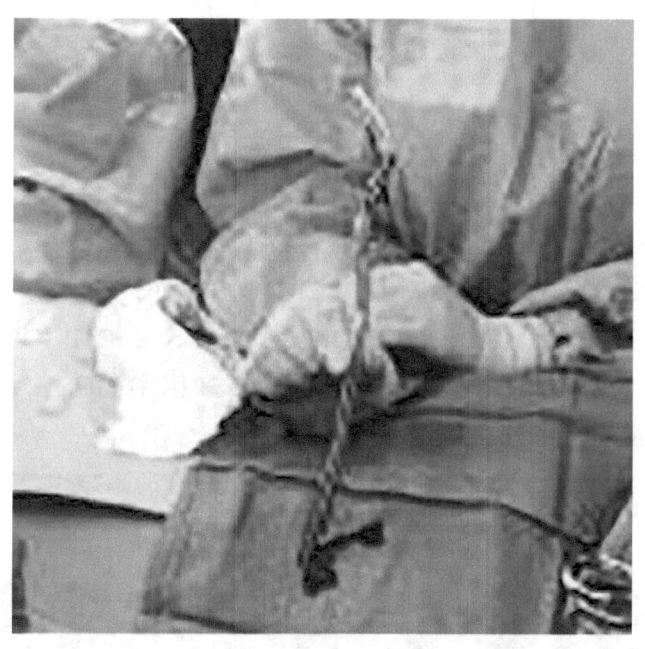

Arrow pointing at removed chest tube

Knowing she was from Scotland, I surmised she was a big football (soccer) fan. There are two competing teams from the 1800s, the Glasgow Rangers and Celtic. I took a fifty-fifty chance and wore my Glasgow Rangers kit to see her the following morning in the ICU. She immediately beamed, as she was a die-hard Rangers fan; she called her family in Scotland to tell them she was being cared for by a Rangers doctor. She was discharged home to Scotland, a very lucky lady indeed to have survived the incident. The ER doctor should have gotten a better history from the patient.

Chapter 11

A forty-three-year-old man was referred to the thoracic clinic by his bariatric surgeon. Two years prior, he had a lap band placed for weight loss. Over that time, he had worsening chest tightness, difficulty swallowing, and malodorous breath. He was found to have a large 8 by 7 cm. intrathoracic esophageal diverticulum (outpouching).

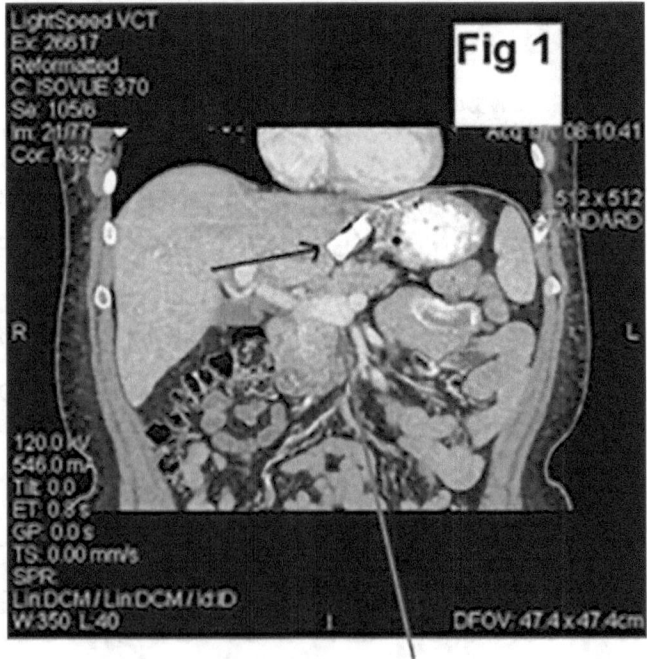

Arrow pointing to lap band

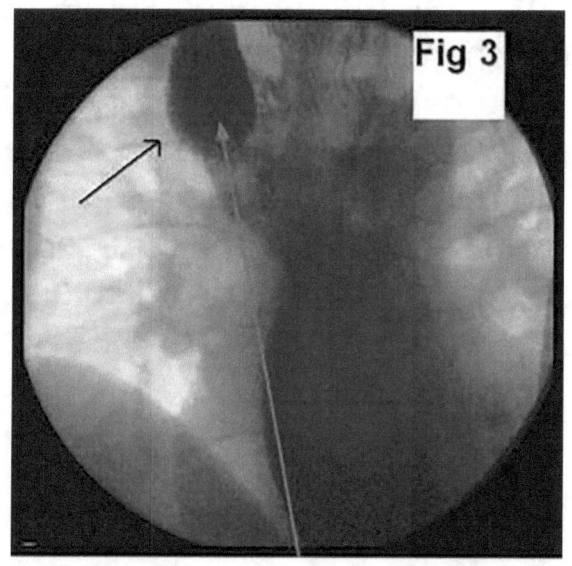

Barium contrast swallow arrow pointing to diverticulum

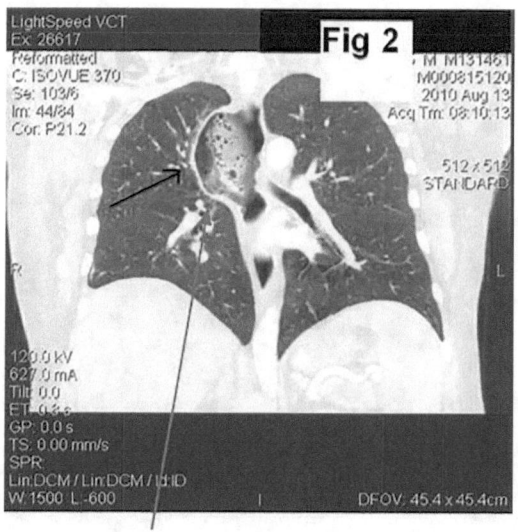

Arrow pointing to diverticulum

We opted for surgical management to resect the diverticulum. First, the bariatric surgeon removed the lap band, then we opened the chest and stapled the diverticulum. On post-op day two, his barium swallow showed a good passage of the contrast with no leak. I surmised that the lap band increased pressure on the esophagus and the esophagus then ballooned, thus forming the diverticulum.

Chapter 12

Collision Tumor

A fifty-five-year-old man presented with a fungating 20 cm. lesion on his left shoulder cheat area. He had a history of nontreated AIDS and did not seek care for his necrotic skin lesion. The lesion was ulcerated, foul smelling, necrotic, and infested with maggots. He was very ill and was admitted to the hospital. We were consulted and recommended operative biopsies and assess possible resection. In the OR, we eradicated the maggots with the betadine prep; I visualized that there seemed to be two distinct tumor architectures, with a collision of the tumors in the center. He was deemed nonresectable, but we biopsied, and sure enough, two distinct tumor types were verified by pathology.

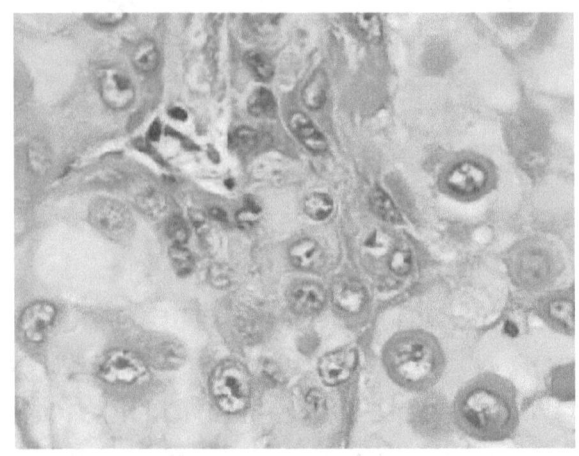

Squamous cell

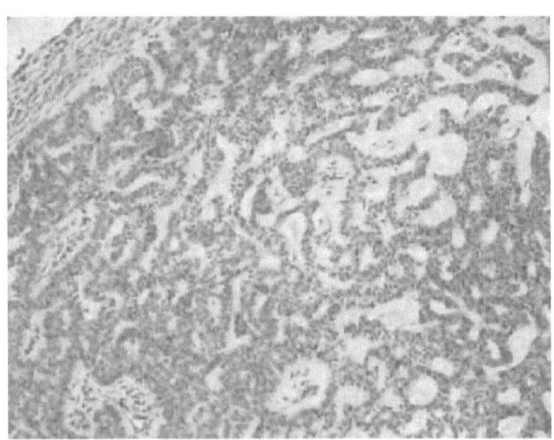

Basal cell

The pathologist reported two distinct cancers: basal cell and squamous cell. The tumors collided in the center of the lesion. Unfortunately, he did not do well and was discharged to hospice. Collision tumors are very rare comprising only 1 percent of soft tissue cancers.

Chapter 13
Pseudosarcoma

A fifty-four-year-old morbidly obese African American with an extensive past medical history of sleep-disordered breathing managed on BiPAP at home, poorly controlled diabetes, anemia, and lower extremity cellulitis with lymphedema. The patient presented for the evaluation of a huge mass of the right leg, complaining of a gradual increase in size and weight of the mass, hence affecting his mobility and quality of life.

He had stated significant complications with activities of daily living, walking, gait, and balance and back pain that had chronically worsened with increasing the size of the mass.

The physical exam showed a morbidly obese man with a pedunculated mass of the medial proximal right thigh and lower extremity edema. CT scan of the mass interpreted the mass as "large (33 cm. x 27 cm.) minimally heterogeneously enhancing soft tissue mass arising from the subcutaneous tissues of medial right thigh containing area of fat attenuation-differentiated liposarcoma should be considered as well as other benign and malignant soft tissue tumors."

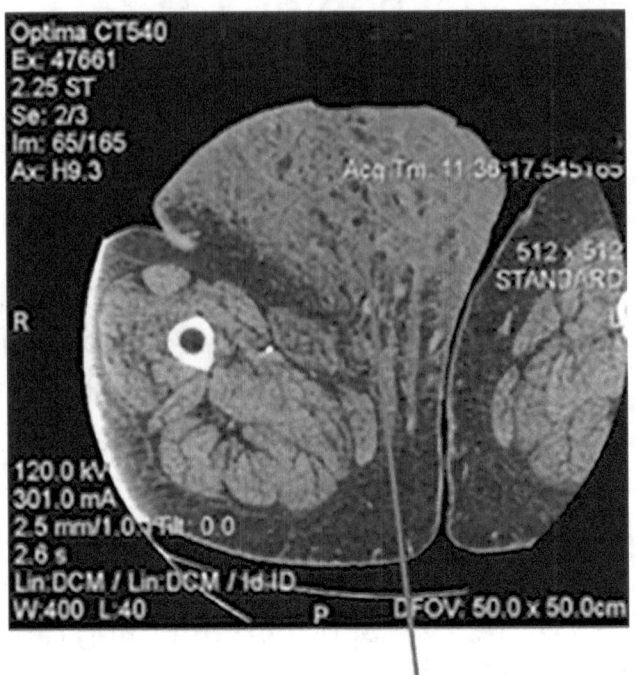

CT scan thigh mass

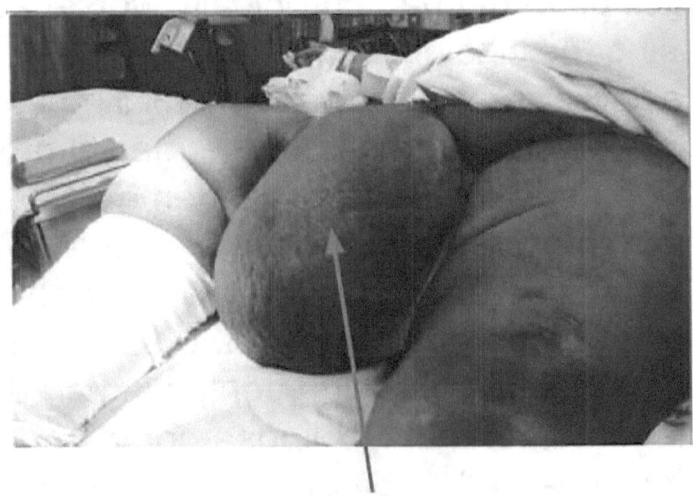

Thigh mass

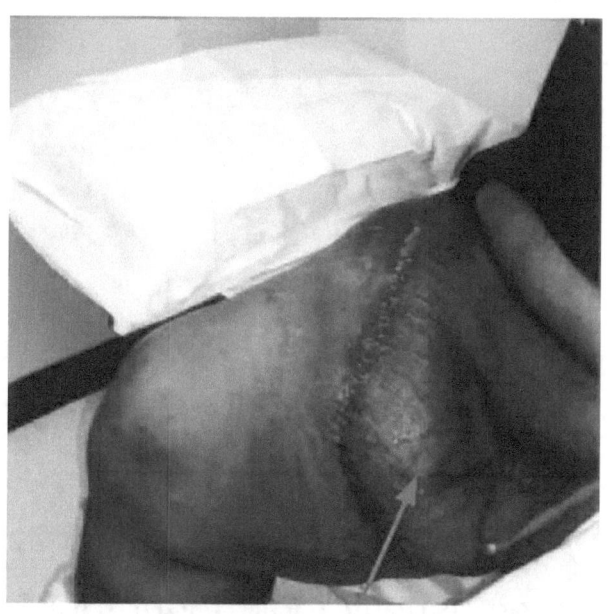

Six weeks post-op

The mass measured 49 cm. by 30 cm. by 13 cm. and weighed 39.6 kg.; final diagnosis is localized lymphedema (pseudosarcoma). He did well and was able to start exercising, his initial weight was 535 pounds, and he lost about one hundred pounds in the first year. We completed four additional cases over the next year with great success. Unfortunately, may surgeons have avoided such cases; they are complex. The blood vessels feeding such tumors are massive, and the lymphatic channels are robust. We used innovative techniques including the Aquamantys cautery and used superheated water to cut and cauterize the vessels.

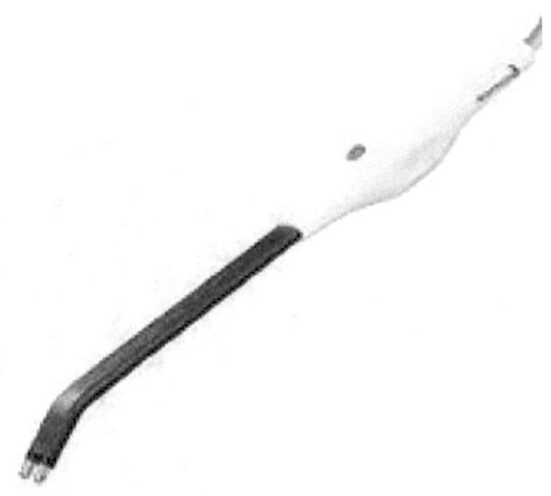

The cases usually took about four hours; all patients needed wound vac closure of the large defect after resection. Wounds took 4–8 months to heal. The patients were able to ambulate and increase mobility after losing an eighty-five-pound tumor. Their quality of life markedly improved as well.

Chapter 14
Pulmonary Hernia

A fifty-nine-year-old man with increased body habitus and no previous history of trauma or rib fractures, thoracic operations, COPD, tobacco use, and/or corticosteroid use presented to our clinic endorsing a prior one-week history of bacterial pneumonia. The patient was seen by three physicians over a six-month period prior to being properly referred to our team. His past medical history was significant for hypertension, myocardial infarction, coronary artery disease with numerous angioplasties, and gastroesophageal reflux disease. While ill with the prior pneumonia infection, the patient endured a forceful coughing spell lasting approximately three minutes in duration. During this spell, he experienced a popping and tearing sensation in his right thorax followed by a sharp pain in the lower right aspect of his chest wall. After the incident, he described a baseline of low-intensity dull pain, with transient exacerbations of severe pain. Inspection of the right hemithorax revealed a widening of the eighth intercostal space, with a mass appreciated from posterior- to anterior axillary line during the Valsalva maneuver. The mass was tender and reducible.

Chest radiography and computed tomography revealed protrusion of the air-containing right lung and inferolateral right chest wall through the right lateral eighth intercostal space. No rib fractures, effusions, and pneumothorax were noted on evaluation of imaging.

A right thoracotomy with pulmonary hernia repair was performed. There was a significant diastasis noted at the right eighth intercostal space. Prior to closure, a 20-French chest drain was placed through an inferior interspace. Primary closure of the defect and ribs was conducted. No mesh was used in this operation. The patient's recovery was uneventful, and he was discharged home on postoperative day number three. At follow-up, the incision site had healed nicely with no recurrence and the patient did not endorse any physical complaints from his surgical intervention.

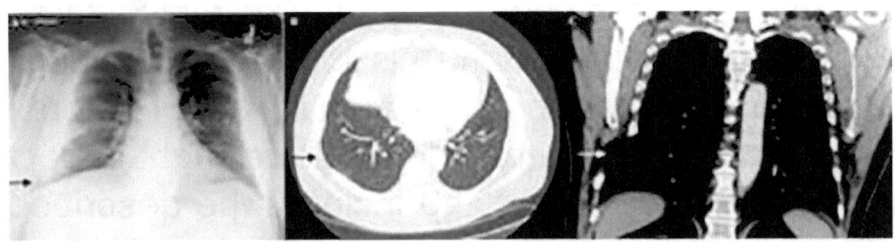

Chest radiograph (A) and computed tomography (B and C) revealing protrusion of the air containing right lung along with the inferolateral right chest wall at the right lateral eighth intercostal space

SLIPH (spontaneous lateral intercostal pulmonary hernias) is extremely rare and may occur in individuals with very few modifiable and nonmodifiable risk factors. There appears to be less than a dozen reported true cases of SLIPH in the literature. This case is unique as it appears to be the only presentation of SLIPH secondary to pneumonia.

Chapter 15

I hope you enjoyed the previous, most interesting cases. As you probably surmised, I miss the operating room and the ability to help patients that other surgeons have avoided. It's a wonderful feeling to see the results and how their lives are improved. This was the case with diagnosing the first xiphoid syndrome. To recall, she was a sixteen-year-old high school basketball player who was out of breath, had pain in the shoulders and back, and was unable to play the sport she loved. Prior to her consultation with us, she saw twelve doctors, who were all mystified, and many recommended antipsychotics. She was referred to our clinic; I diagnosed the problem as her xiphoid. And the rest is history. She had a rapid recovery and got back on the team; they clinched not one but two state championships. She went on to play basketball on a college scholarship.

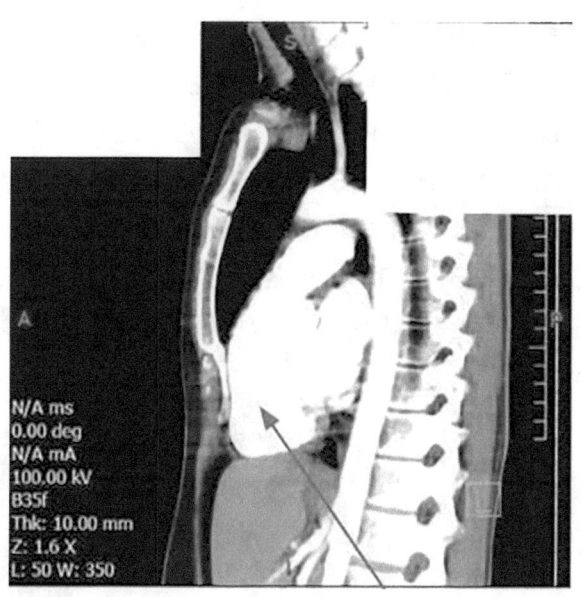

Arrow pointing at xiphoid, pressing on the heart

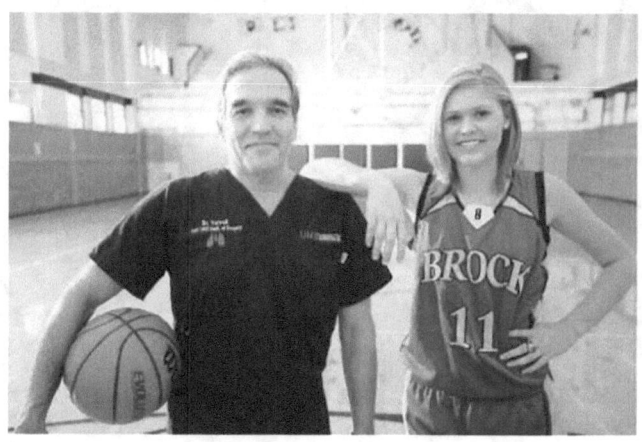

Following her case, we received lots of press and the patients started coming from all over the country. Notable was a fantastic musician, Zakk, from Colorado; his recovery was remarkable, his band has opened for many artists, he has produced music videos, and I believe one day he will receive a Grammy. We also had international patients, one from Canada and one from the Netherlands. The Netherlands case was a Royal Marine who, as a sniper, lies on his chest, causing severe pain around the xiphoid area, which was affecting his accuracy. He returned to active duty and reported he was "back on target."

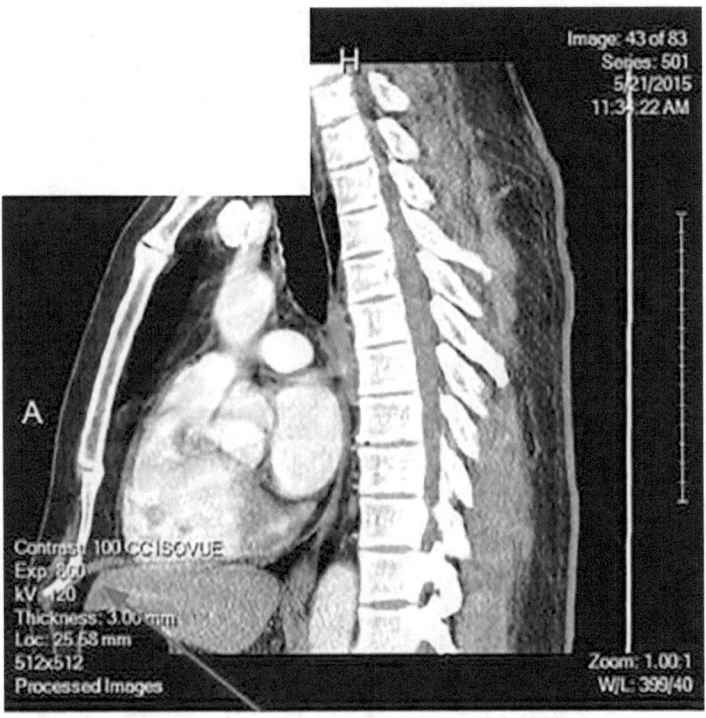

Arrow pointing to the xiphoid

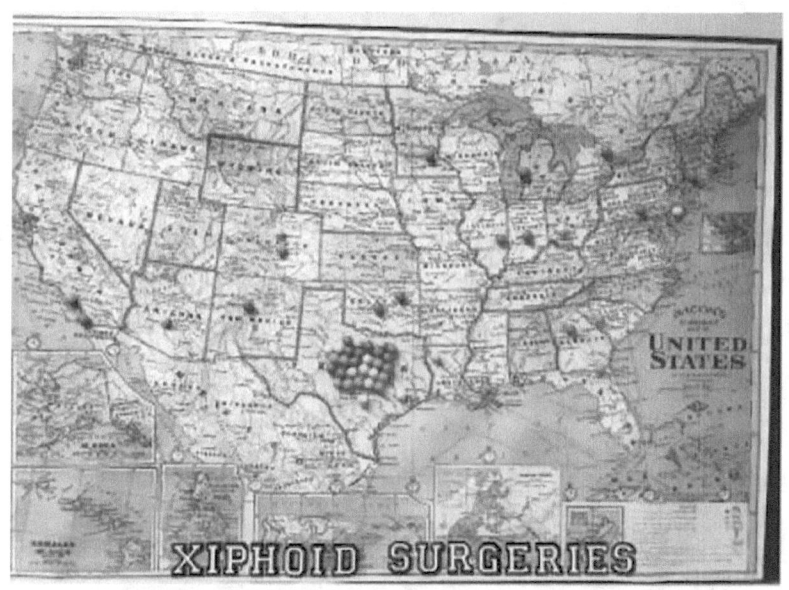

Initial map of xiphoid referrals

This map was displayed in our clinic; patients placed a pin on the map indicating where they were from. We initially published the largest series in *International Surgery*. By the time I had to give up surgery, we had completed ninety-six xiphoid resections. I still receive emails from around the country asking for help; unfortunately, I cannot help them, and it saddens me. I have not been able to engage any thoracic surgeon to take up the challenge.

Chapter 16

So the Fates have interfered again! I developed Cushing's syndrome, secondary to steroids. This syndrome is illustrated in a series of books by a physician artist Frank Netter, MD.

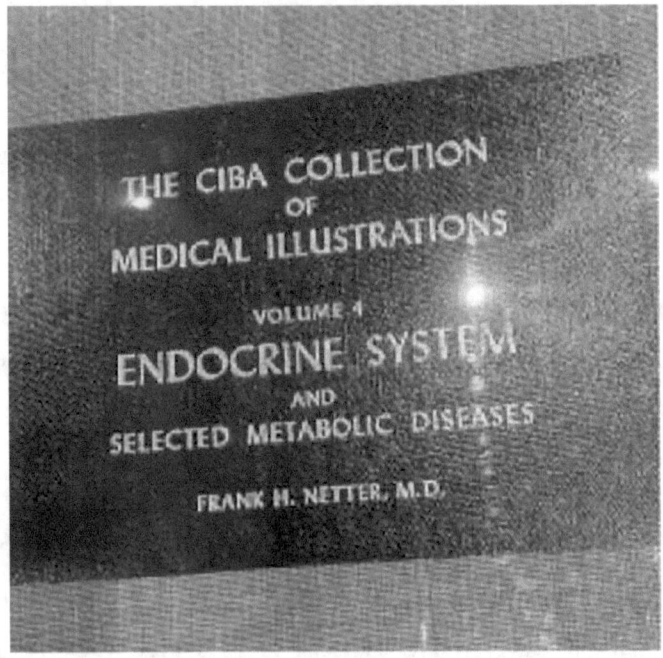

THE CIBA COLLECTION
OF
MEDICAL ILLUSTRATIONS

VOLUME 4

ENDOCRINE SYSTEM
AND
SELECTED METABOLIC DISEASES

FRANK H. NETTER, M.D.

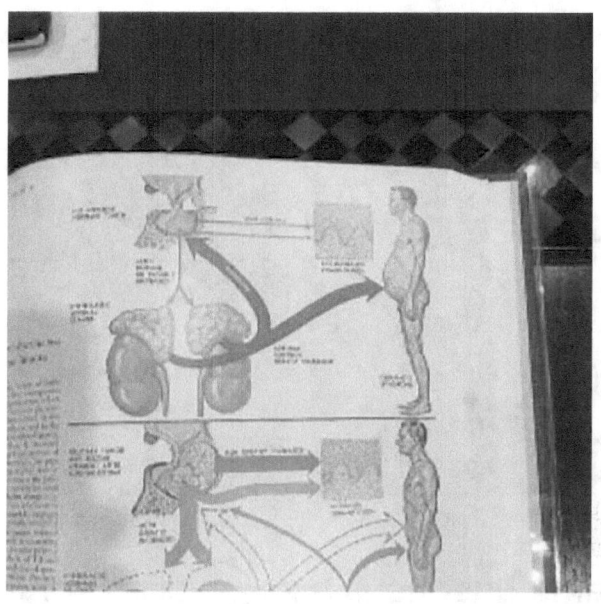

In his books are illustrated explanations of a patient with Cushing's syndrome. I am a poster boy: moon face, belly, and weight gain. So what exactly is Cushing's syndrome?

In 1932, American neurosurgeon Harvey Cushing described the clinical findings that provided the link between specific physical characteristics (e.g., abnormal obesity of the face and trunk) and a specific type of pituitary tumor. This pituitary disorder became known as Cushing syndrome. Cushing's syndrome is a rare endocrine illness caused by exposure of body tissues to too much cortisol in the bloodstream. Produced by the adrenal glands, cortisol is a substance (hormone) that helps the body control blood pressure and respond to stress. Extra cortisol, however, produces abnormal body changes.

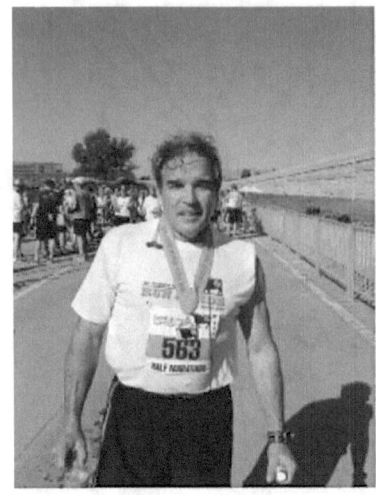 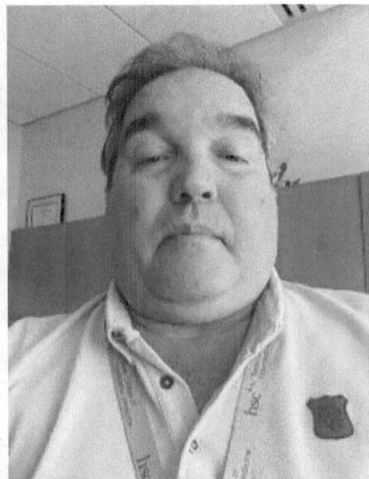

Presteroids   Poststeroids

Dexamethasone is a long-acting corticosteroid that is about twenty five times more potent (stronger) than hydrocortisone and six times more potent than prednisone. For reference, your body naturally makes the equivalent of about 5 mg. of prednisone daily. My endocrinologist has tried to substitute hydrocortisone, but the substitution has not been therapeutic.

As you gain weight, you now develop insulin resistance and elevated blood sugars; steroids will also increase your blood glucose. This puts you at risk for type 2 diabetes.

So the Fates are back, and sure enough, I developed diabetes! I did not realize my glucose was in the 200-plus range; normal is 90–110, which explains weight gain and other symptoms.

As usual, insurance companies do not want to pay for the monitor or the injectable; a one-month course of therapy is $900 without insurance. We were able to receive authorization for an injectable at a $100 copay per month.

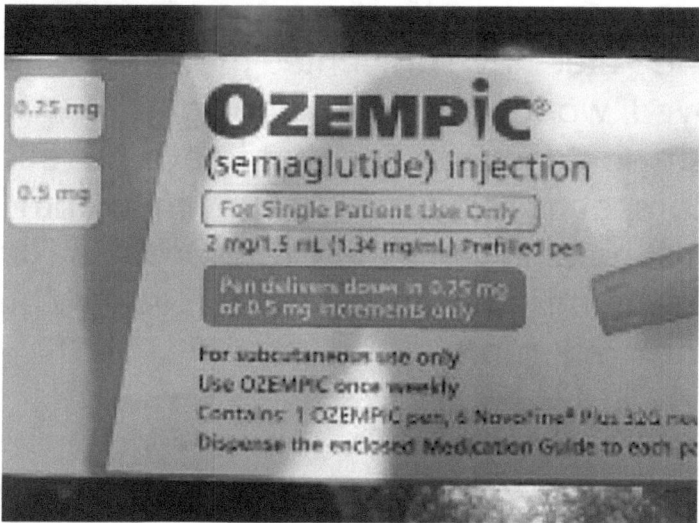

Thanks to the Fates, I have another disease to deal with, diabetes. I now have a continuous glucose monitoring device, a fascinating technology that allows you to check your blood glucose in real time. Hope we can get my HbA1c down to a normal range.

Chapter 17

So the Fates have prevented me from doing what I enjoyed, working out and running.

I am so deconditioned that I have no reserve. I was competing in a run almost every month.

Most notable were the Great Scottish Run and the one-hundredth anniversary Rocky Mountain National Park run.

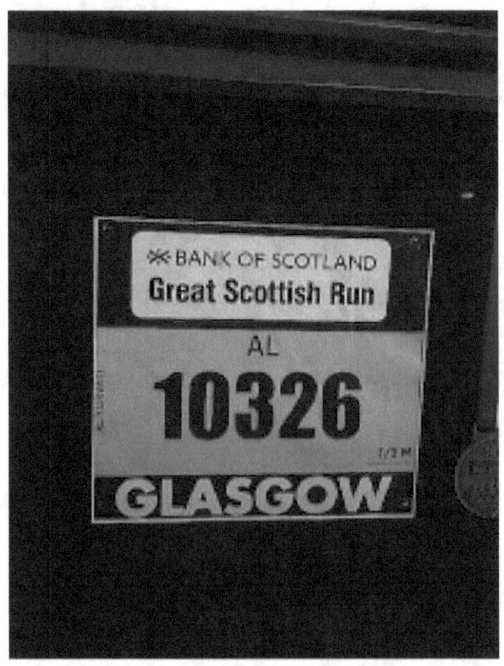

Great Scottish Run, Glasgow, Scotland, 2013

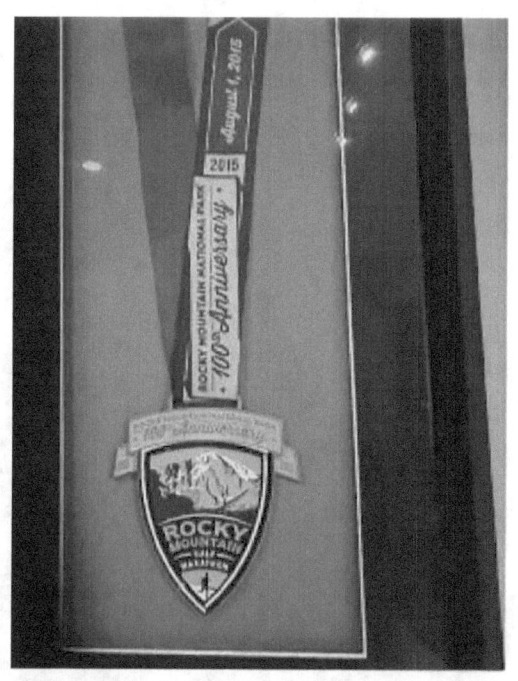

Rocky Mountain National Park one-hundredth anniversary, 2015

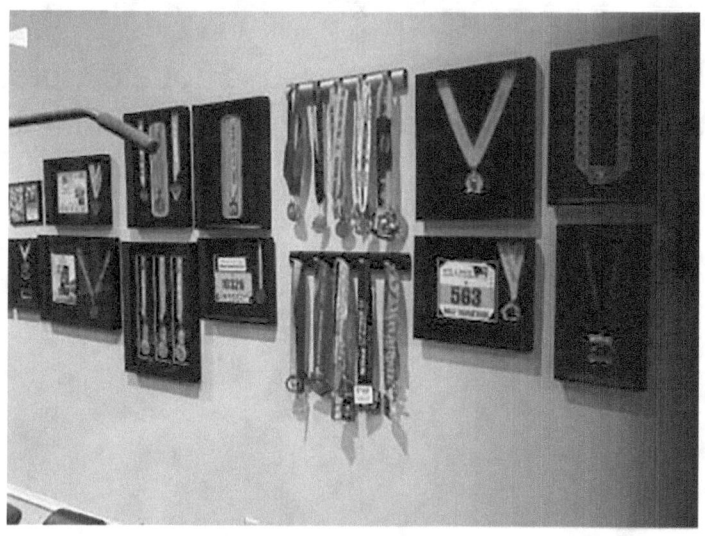

Finisher medals

Also, I was bodybuilding and weight lifting; my maximum bench press was 340 pounds. I am lucky if I could bench press five pounds. The Fates have it in for me!

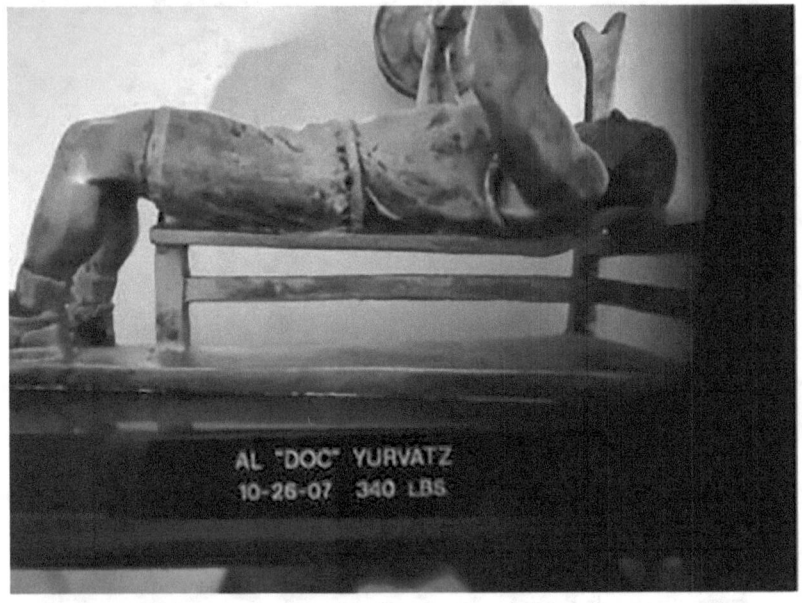

AL "DOC" YURVATZ
10-26-07 340 LBS

Well, I just need to start slow and hopefully progress. With all the spine hardware, my flexibility is gone.

Chapter 18

One of the most rewarding things that the Fates have given me was the ability to train some stellar students and residents. Notable was Dr. Morgan, who I first met as a TCOM student in my honors class "Historical Aspects of Cardiac Surgery." She was a general surgery resident with us at Medical City Fort Worth, then went on to do a trauma fellowship at the University of Alabama; she is now a trauma surgeon in Plano, Texas. Dr. Thomas was a surgery resident with us and also did a trauma fellowship. Dr. Ron was the same, but he did a third fellowship in hand surgery. All are excellent surgeons and board certified.

I had the honor of hooding all three of my former residents as fellows of the American College of Osteopathic Surgeons. I occasionally receive messages from them on how they applied techniques I taught them and have saved patients; it's a fantastic feeling, the transfer of knowledge.

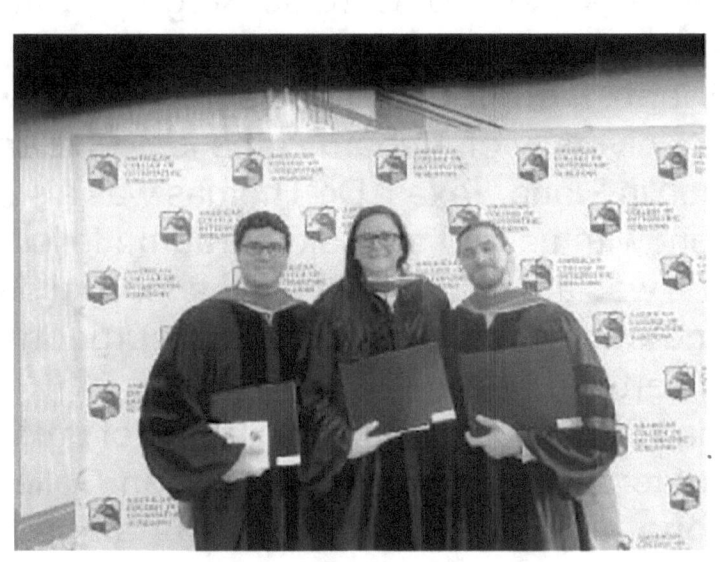

Chapter 19

I hope you enjoyed book two, "*This to Me.*" The title comes from our chief of cardiac surgery, Dr. LBM; at the start of a case, he would say, "This to me," and the scrub tech would hand him the scalpel. This was before the current time-out in surgery; he was ahead of time!

I am contemplating book three, revisiting topics/ sites with new pictures; I plan to title book three "*30 Degrees on Bypass.*" So stay tuned as the Fates are still interfering with my life.

All proceeds from royalties go to the TCOM General Student Scholarship as well as the University of Strathclyde General Student Scholarship. So if the book is rubbish, at least buy a copy to help out the students.

About the Author

Albert H. Yurvati, DO, PhD, DFACOS, FICS, FAHA, is a 1986 graduate of the Texas College of Osteopathic Medicine at the University of North Texas Health Science Center. He completed his internship and general surgery residency at Tulsa Regional Medical Center in Tulsa, Oklahoma, and served as chief resident in his final year. He then completed a residency in cardiothoracic and vascular surgery at the Deborah Heart and Lung Center in Robert Wood Johnson Medical School at Browns Mills, New Jersey, where he also served as chief resident.

He is AOA board certified in cardiothoracic-vascular and general surgery, and he is a fellow of the American College of Surgeons as well as the International College of Surgeons. He was one of the inaugural Distinguished Fellows of the American College of Osteopathic Surgeons.

He completed a PhD in education with a concentration on organizational leadership from Northcentral University. Other educational activities include a graduate certificate from the University of North Texas Toulouse School of Education in teaching and adult learning.

Currently, Dr. Yurvati is a tenured DSWOP professor of surgery and chair of the Department of

Medical Education at the Texas College of Osteopathic Medicine, and he is a professor of integrative physiology at the Institute of Cardiovascular and Metabolic Disease. He is a visiting professor at the University of Strathclyde in Glasgow, Scotland, in the Department of Biomedical Engineering.

He has received numerous awards from the UNTHSC, including the 2012 Clyde Gallehugh DO Memorial Award and the 2011 President's Award for Clinical Excellence. He also received Doctor of Philanthropy in 2011, and in 2010, he was the recipient of both the Benjamin L. Cohen Award for Outstanding Research Achievement and the TCOM's Dean's Award for Philanthropy. In addition, he received the Academic Commendation of Excellence (ACE) Award for superior posttenure review.

On a national level, Dr. Yurvati was the executive director of the American Osteopathic Board of Surgery. He is actively involved in numerous committees of the ACOS, and he has served as a discipline chair and representative to the board of governors as well as a cardiothoracic educational program director. In 2013, he received the highest award from the American College of Osteopathic Surgeons: the Orel F. Martin Medal. In 2016, he received the ACOS Guy D. Beaumont Education Award.

He is on the editorial board of multiple journals, including the JAOA and Filtration. He is a reviewer for many peered journals to include *Cardiovascular*

Research, Experimental Biology and Medicine, the Annals of Thoracic Surgery, and the JAOA. Dr. Yurvati has published over one hundred peer-reviewed articles, three book chapters, and numerous abstracts. He is the recipient of over 2.5 million in grants, including NIH, NASA, DOD, and Osteopathic Heritage Foundation funding. He has lectured nationally and internationally. Dr. Yurvati is the associate designated institutional official for the Medical City Healthcare Consortium's ACGME-accredited programs. He also served on the ACGME working group for Surgery Milestones 2.0.